My
MENTAL HEALTH
MEDICATION
WORKBOOK

My MENTAL HEALTH MEDICATION WORKBOOK

FRAN MILLER, RN, MSN, BC

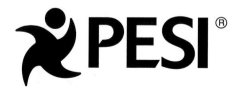 PESI®

EAU CLAIRE, WISCONSIN

2006

PESI, LLC
PO Box 1000
200 Spring Street
Eau Claire, Wisconsin 54702

Printed in the United States of America

ISBN: 0-9749711-8-9

PESI, LLC strives to obtain knowledgeable authors and faculty for its publications and seminars. The clinical recommendations contained herein are the result of extensive author research and review. Obviously, any recommendations for patient care must be held up against individual circumstances at hand. To the best of our knowledge any recommendations included by the author or faculty reflect currently accepted practice. However, these recommendations cannot be considered universal and complete. The authors and publisher repudiate any responsibility for unfavorable effects that result from information, recommendations, undetected omissions or errors. Professionals using this publication should research other original sources of authority as well.

For information on this and other PESI manuals and
audio recordings, please call 800-843-7763 or
visit our website at www.pesi.com

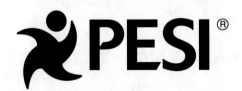

SAM011565 9/06

Table of Contents

Introduction

Emotional symptoms affect many people of all ages. It is estimated that 1 out of every 6 people experience some form of mental illness in their lifetime. These symptoms affect your ability to cope with daily life as well as managing stressful situations.

When emotional symptoms become too painful or get out of control, they are referred to as psychiatric symptoms. It is really important for you to seek professional treatment. Psychiatric treatment usually includes counseling as well as taking medication.

The use of medication in psychiatric treatment has become a critical part of recovery and essential in the prevention of *relapse*. Relapse is a term that refers to the return of your symptoms. Recent knowledge of the brain including biological causes of mental illness has made recovery possible. Medication can help a person to recover and lead a normal life. Mental health medications are now viewed as essential for complete brain health.

Relapse can be a very painful and demoralizing experience. When you stop taking your medication, your risk of relapse is 5 times higher. It will take longer to recover. Your medication may not work as well. You may need higher doses of your medication, which could increase the risks of annoying side effects. Many times a person is unable to return to their previous level of functioning. This could result in the loss of a job, family, friends, and even housing.

In spite of this knowledge, medication *noncompliance*, or not taking the medication as prescribed, continues to be a major problem for mental health patients. It is estimated that 10% of all hospitalizations may be due to medication noncompliance. It may lead to loss of income due to missed work days. It is estimated that 50% *of all medications used* are not taken correctly. Some research studies of patients taking mental health medications report only taking them 20–40% of the time.

Purpose of this Workbook

This workbook is written to provide you with a better understanding of your illness and how medications help to treat your symptoms. It teaches you the necessary steps to take for mental health recovery. Having an understanding of your mental illness and symptoms is the first step towards wellness. This workbook takes you step by step on the road to recovery. It is specifically designed for you to use with your doctor and other members of your treatment team. By using this workbook, you will able to better understand your illness and how to manage your recovery.

The following list covers key points that you may want to know and learn about your illness. You may want to begin this process by discussing these key points with your treatment team. Medication compliance and recovery is a collaborative effort between you and your doctor/nurse practitioner, and your counselor. The groups of professionals you work with are referred to as your treatment team.

What I Should Know About My Mental Illness and My Medications

1. My symptoms and diagnosis
2. Factors that contributed to my symptoms
3. The possible chemical transmission problems in my brain
4. My treatment options including counseling/education as well as medications
5. The names of my medications
6. The purpose of my medications
7. How to take my medications
8. The side effects of my medications and how to deal with them
9. How to monitor my progress
10. What will happen if I drink or use "street" drugs

Why Am I Having Symptoms?

How my brain works

Your brain is the hardware of your soul according to Daniel Amen MD.[1] It determines what you think and perceive, how you feel, and how you interact with others. When you are depressed, angry, or confused, you may think it is just an emotional problem.

Brain Diagram

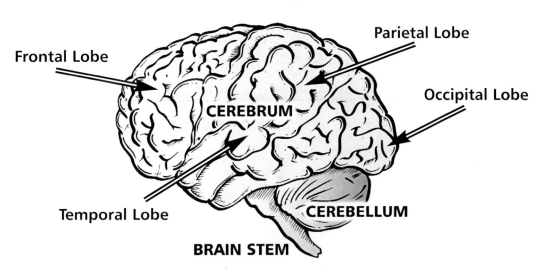

In reality, your brain's ability to function plays an important role in all your thoughts and feelings. Your brain manufactures chemicals that convert into thoughts and feelings. It is "hardwired" with brain cells. Each part of your brain plays a specific role in processing and storing information

Brain cells, which are called neurons, are lined up in order to pass messages from one cell to another. They do not touch each other, so they are unable to pass the message directly. These chemicals in your brain that carry messages are called *neurotransmitters*.

Each neuron has three major parts. The *dendrite* receives the message. And the *cell body* is the command center and contains your unique "blueprint" referred to as DNA for interpreting the information. The *axon* consists of fibers that prepare the message to be sent on to the next neuron. The space between each neuron is called the *synapse*. The axon releases the "message carriers" or neurotransmitters into the synapse and carries the information to the dendrites of the next neuron. The dendrite is like tree branches. Messages must attach to a specific spot of a specific branch. Once the message is attached to the next dendrite, the neurotransmitters return home to the axon by via a "reuptake pump."

1   Amen, Daniel, MD, *Change Your Brain, Change Your Life,* page 3, 1998

Neuron Diagram

Dendrite: receives the message

Cell body: the command center where your DNA affects the interpretation of the message

Axon: sends the message on the next neuron

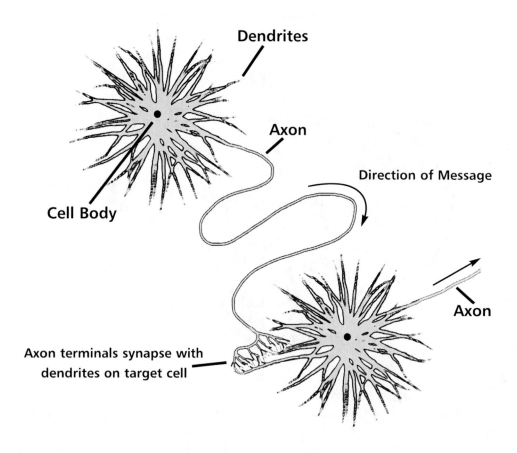

There are more than 100 billion neurons in your brain with 100 trillion connecting pathways between them. The connections are made by electrical impulses carried by chemical messengers that transmit from neuron to neuron.

Your brain produces over 100,000 chemical reactions in any given second. They work like a radio transmitter to send specific messages to a specific place. It is similar to the global phone network. You dial one number and only one phone rings.

There are many types of chemicals that are manufactured in the brain. Certain chemicals function as "messagers" or neurotransmitters by working in the synaptic space between each neuron. Neurotransmitters carry the message and attach it to the appropriate place on the dendrite of the next neuron. When all the parts and functions of the brain are working correctly, your thoughts and feelings are accurate and functional.

Messages travel specific pathways or highways depending on the type of message or signal. These pathways are a part of special processing places or systems in the brain. They not only process the message, they store the information for future use.

Diagram of Brain Systems

The following diagram identifies the primary systems of the brain and where they are located:

Limbic System: sets your emotional tones

Basal Ganglia: stores patterns of behavior

Prefrontal Cortex: most evolved part of the brain allows you to do abstract thinking and learning, decision-making, and problem solving

Cingulate Systems: allows you to shift attention

Temporal Lobes: stores memories & experiences

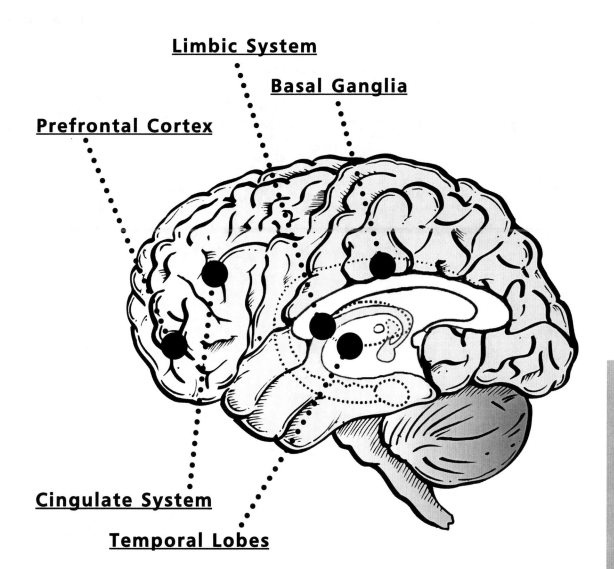

11

What happens when brain chemicals get out of balance?

Symptoms are related to errors in chemical messaging. If there are problems in the transmission, your brain will signal with emotional symptoms like anxiety or depression. You could also experience problems with concentration, thinking, problem-solving, or relating to others. The brain chemical transmission system receives only bits and pieces of information. Your brain struggles to fit the pieces together. Your limbic system "overworks" and produces the emotional symptoms. These symptoms help to determine your psychiatric diagnosis.

When there is not enough or too much chemical messaging between neurons, your symptoms will occur. This problem sometimes is referred to as having a chemical imbalance in your brain.

Diagram of Chemical Transmission

Diagram A shows the chemical transmission of brain cells that are working effectively.

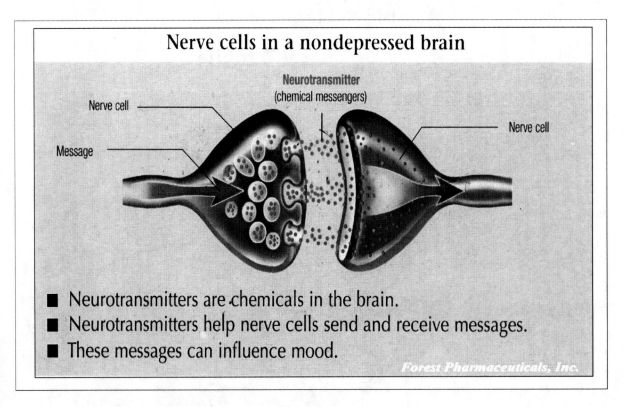

Diagram A

Diagram B shows what happens when the neurotransmitters are not working effectively.

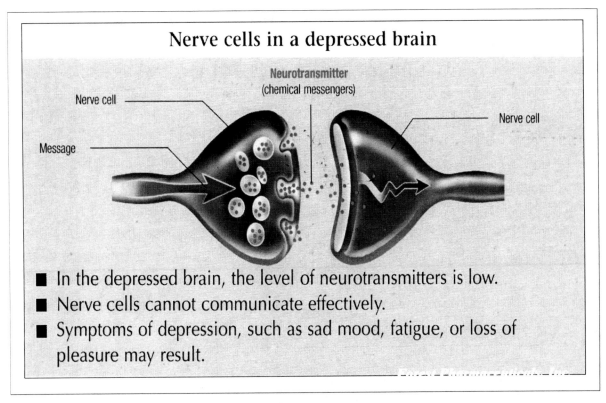

Nerve cells in a depressed brain

Neurotransmitter (chemical messengers)

Nerve cell

Nerve cell

Message

■ In the depressed brain, the level of neurotransmitters is low.
■ Nerve cells cannot communicate effectively.
■ Symptoms of depression, such as sad mood, fatigue, or loss of pleasure may result.

Diagram B

How does my medication work in my brain?

Psychiatric medications primarily work to correct the problems with the chemical messaging systems in your brain, which is referred to as neurotransmission. They may help by adjusting the balance of chemical "messagers." Some of the medications work to increase the amount of neurotransmission. Some medications work to block the neurotransmission when there is too much getting in the connecting brain cell. Every dose of medicine works to balance the neurotransmission system. If you stop taking the medication, the imbalance will return.

Chemicals in my brain that affect emotion

The chemicals, or neurotransmitters, in the brain that seem to be related to mood are Dopamine, Serotonin, and Norepinephrine. They all seem to relate to mood but each has their own uniqueness. The following diagram helps to define their uniqueness:

NEUROTRANSMITTERS

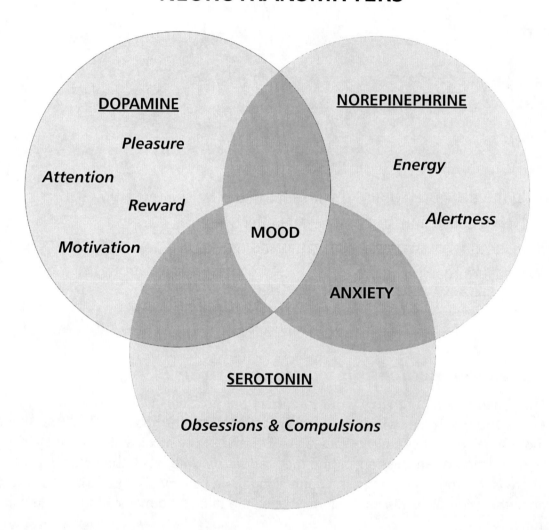

14

Dopamine affects your ability to experience pleasure; helps your mood; helps with motivation and energy; helps you think, concentrate and be social.

Serotonin helps you be calm and in a good mood; helps you sleep.

Norepinephrine helps alertness, working memory, concentration, information processing and problem-solving; helps mood and fatigue.

What Makes My Symptoms Worse?

There may be factors in your life that can worsen your symptoms or interfere in your recovery. You may need to make changes in your daily living activities that will help to hasten your recovery from your mental illness. These common factors are:

- *When I don't get treatment*

    Your symptoms can be very painful and upsetting, but they are very important. They are the signals that tell you to get treatment. Your symptoms will most likely worsen if they are not treated. Find a health care provider that you are comfortable with and see them as soon as possible.

- *When I have difficulty with coping with stress*

    Sometimes you have too many problems at one time. This can be very overwhelming. Feelings like anxiety and frustration will worsen. You will probably experience difficulty concentrating, loss of sleep and loss of energy. Your ability to cope becomes greatly diminished.

- *When I have problems with relationships*

    Your relationships with your family members, loved ones, friends, or co-workers are very important and have a major impact on how you feel. If you are having problems with others, the stress of those problems will increase your painful feelings and symptoms.

- *When I am not leading a healthy lifestyle*

    Proper diet, adequate exercise and restful sleep are essential to emotional and physical health. If you are not getting appropriate amounts of each, your energy is lessened, your frustration tolerance is compromised, and your ability to concentrate is diminished. Your ability to cope and function will decrease and your symptoms will likely increase.

    List the factors that may interfere in your recovery.

1. _____

2. _____

3. _____

How Do I Get Relief from My Symptoms?

Recognizing my symptoms

Recognizing your symptoms is one of the first steps in getting relief from your symptoms. Your symptoms usually include problems with:

- Increased anxiety and painful feelings.

- Problems with managing your emotions.

- Problems with concentration, problem-solving, and thinking.

- Increased physical problems.

- Increased difficulty managing your life activities and relationships.

Understanding my symptoms

Another important step is to understand that having emotional problems or a mental illness is considered a medical illness. You wonder why this has happened to you. Like other medical problems, there may be many contributing factors. Some of these factors are genetic and some are environmental.

You should not blame yourself or others or feel ashamed that you have the problem. Just like having a heart attack, you did not plan on it. It can be treated, it does not have to be fatal, and you will be able to participate in a treatment program to recover and return to normal functioning.

How Can I Get Relief from My Symptoms?

In order to get relief from your symptoms, you will need to take medication and learn to develop healthier coping skills. Your treatment providers may require you to participate in both of the following:

16

1. Attend counseling sessions to help to understand your illness, improve your coping skills, learn more effective problem-solving and stress management.

2. Take medication, monitor your progress, and attend your medication management appointments.

Understanding My Illness and Psychiatric Diagnosis

Understanding your illness and how to treat your symptoms is important for symptom relief. The next step is to have your Doctor help determine your psychiatric diagnosis.

The following common psychiatric diagnoses can impact your ability to function and carry out your activities in daily living. Your relationships with others can also be problematic due to your symptoms.

The common psychiatric diagnoses include:

1. Depression
2. Anxiety (Panic Disorder)
3. Mood Disorder (Bipolar Disorder)
4. Post Traumatic Stress Disorder (PTSD)
5. Emotion Regulation Problems
6. Attention Deficit Disorder (ADHD)
7. Cognitive Impairment (MCI, Dementia)
8. Psychotic Disorder (Schizophrenia)

In the next few pages you will find examples of symptoms that are common to a specific mental health problem. Each problem category can be considered a psychiatric diagnosis.

Please select the psychiatric diagnosis that best describes your primary symptoms.

1. Indicate which of the common symptoms you have.
2. List any additional symptoms.
3. Indicate the approximate date the symptoms started. (month or week).
4. Indicate the frequency of your symptoms.
5. The "changes in frequency" column may be used after you have initiated medication to report any changes or improvements.
6. If your symptoms seem to fit more than one diagnosis, you can utilize any that apply.

Depression

Depression is a serious medical condition. It is more than feeling "blue" or "down in the dumps" for a few days. It is feeling "down" and "low" and "hopeless" for weeks at a time. Depression may include to following symptoms:

- Sad, tearful mood
- Difficulty sleeping and eating
- Not wanting to be around others; "short fuse"
- Increased irritability; fatigue, and loss of motivation
- Loss of interest or pleasure in the activities you once enjoyed
- Difficulty concentrating
- Low self-esteem
- Feelings of hopelessness

My Symptoms	When they started	Frequency (circle)	Changes in frequency
I feel sad, blue, or unhappy		1 2 3 4	
I can't concentrate		1 2 3 4	
I feel tired and have no energy		1 2 3 4	
I feel uneasy, restless, or irritable		1 2 3 4	
I have a "short fuse"		1 2 3 4	
I have trouble sleeping		1 2 3 4	
I eat too little or too much		1 2 3 4	
I have lost interest in many things I used to enjoy		1 2 3 4	
I have trouble making decisions		1 2 3 4	
I feel worthless or have guilt for no reason		1 2 3 4	
I want to die, or kill/hurt myself		1 2 3 4	
(Other Symptoms)		1 2 3 4	
		1 2 3 4	
		1 2 3 4	

Frequency Scale: 1: never   2: occasionally   3: frequently   4: constantly

Anxiety (Panic Disorder, Social Anxiety Disorder)

Anxiety is a normal reaction to stress. But when it becomes an excessive, irrational dread of everyday situations, it has become a disabling disorder. The symptoms may include:

- Nervous energy.

- Anxious and panic-like feelings.

- Increased worry that can't be controlled.

- Increased physical problems like headaches, dizziness, nausea, and diarrhea.

- Increased heart rate, shortness of breath, chest pain, sweating, trembling or shaking.

- Feelings of unreality or being detached from yourself.

My Symptoms	When they started	Frequency (circle)	Changes in frequency
I worry excessively		1 2 3 4	
I have physical symptoms like shortness of breath, heart palpitations, sweaty palms, nervousness, tremors		1 2 3 4	
I feel like I will lose control		1 2 3 4	
I feel fearful		1 2 3 4	
I am afraid to go places		1 2 3 4	
I have recurrent thoughts		1 2 3 4	
I feel compelled to repeat my actions or behaviors		1 2 3 4	
(Other Symptoms)		1 2 3 4	
		1 2 3 4	
		1 2 3 4	
		1 2 3 4	

Frequency Scale: 1: never   2: occasionally   3: frequently   4: constantly

Mood Disorder (Bipolar Disorder)

Mood Disorder a serious medical illness that causes dramatic shifts in mood. Along with the mood shifts severe changes in energy and behavior can occur. There can be periods of "highs" and "lows" as well as normal times. Some of the behavior changes can include:

- Fluctuations in sleep needs.
- Fluctuations in feelings of hopelessness to inflated self esteem.
- Periods of irritability.
- Periods of severe depression.
- Thoughts of self harm.

My Symptoms	When they started	Frequency (circle)	Changes in frequency
I feel excited		1 2 3 4	
I get upset easily		1 2 3 4	
My thoughts are fast and sometimes race		1 2 3 4	
I have more energy than normal		1 2 3 4	
I don't sleep		1 2 3 4	
I have trouble sitting still		1 2 3 4	
I am easily distracted		1 2 3 4	
I do things I normally don't do, like impulsively spending a lot of money, gambling, drinking, or sexual activity		1 2 3 4	
I have mood swings		1 2 3 4	
I get so depressed, I don't get out of bed or get dressed		1 2 3 4	
(Other Symptoms)		1 2 3 4	
		1 2 3 4	
		1 2 3 4	

Frequency Scale: 1: never   2: occasionally   3: frequently   4: constantly

On the next page is a sample of a Monthly Mood Chart. You will find it very helpful to keep track of your mood changes. (*Check the box for each day of the month that describes your mood for the day.*)

Monthly Mood Chart

Days	1	2	3	4	5	6	7	8	9	10	11	12	13	14	15	16	17	18	19	20	21	22	23	24	25	26	27	28	29	30	31
Elevated Mood																															
Severe Impairment																															
Moderate																															
Mild																															
Normal Mood																															
Mild																															
Moderate																															
Severe Impairment																															
Depressed Mood																															
Medication Taken																															
Hours Slept																															
Anxiety Present																															
Irritability Present																															

Problems Resulting from Traumatic Experiences (PTSD)

PTSD is a serious medical condition that results in persistent, frightening thoughts and memories of a traumatic event like rape, physical, emotional, and sexual abuse, or exposure to a terrifying event. Some symptoms include:

- Feelings of fearfulness, numbness, and high anxiety.

- Sleep problems and or nightmares.

My Symptoms	When they started	Frequency (circle)	Changes in frequency
I persistently relive upsetting events of the past		1 2 3 4	
I have bad dreams, nightmares		1 2 3 4	
I avoid reminders of the traumatic event(s)		1 2 3 4	
I have angry outbursts		1 2 3 4	
I fear for my safety (and the safety of my children)		1 2 3 4	
I have difficulty concentrating		1 2 3 4	
I am moody		1 2 3 4	
I have a lot of anxiety		1 2 3 4	
I feel depressed		1 2 3 4	
(Other Symptoms)		1 2 3 4	
		1 2 3 4	
		1 2 3 4	
		1 2 3 4	

Frequency Scale: 1: never   2: occasionally   3: frequently   4: constantly

Problems with Emotional Control

This type of problem sometimes is referred to personality disorder because it develops over time from faulty learning. Problems of emotional control can lead to serious negative behaviors. Symptoms may include:

- Difficulty in containing anger in a public setting.

- May act impulsively to harm themselves and/or others.

- Inability unable to manage emotional arousal.

- Difficulty working with others and managing conflicts.

My Symptoms	When they started	Frequency (circle)	Changes in frequency
I can't control my anger even in public places		1 2 3 4	
I act impulsively		1 2 3 4	
I have difficulty managing all my emotions		1 2 3 4	
I have difficulty with conflict		1 2 3 4	
I am overly aggressive		1 2 3 4	
I am overly sensitive		1 2 3 4	
I become easily frustrated		1 2 3 4	
I have trouble in relationships		1 2 3 4	
I have trouble getting along with my co-workers or other people		1 2 3 4	
(Other Symptoms)		1 2 3 4	
		1 2 3 4	
		1 2 3 4	
		1 2 3 4	

Frequency Scale: 1: never   2: occasionally   3: frequently   4: constantly

Problems with Attention (ADD, ADHD)

A problem with the ability to concentrate and focus, it is often referred to as ADD or ADHD.

- May cause impaired functioning in multiple settings including:

    Home
    Work
    School
    Relationships with others

- May also cause problems finishing tasks and with becoming easily frustrated.

My Symptoms	When they started	Frequency (circle)	Changes in frequency
I am easily distracted		1 2 3 4	
I have difficulty staying focused		1 2 3 4	
I have difficulty being organized		1 2 3 4	
I am frequently losing things		1 2 3 4	
I am restless, "hyper"		1 2 3 4	
I am impulsive		1 2 3 4	
I can't wait my turn		1 2 3 4	
(Other Symptoms)		1 2 3 4	
		1 2 3 4	
		1 2 3 4	
		1 2 3 4	

Frequency Scale: 1: never   2: occasionally   3: frequently   4: constantly

Problems with Memory
(Mild Cognitive Impairment, Dementia)

A serious medical condition characterized by memory lapses, especially short term memory and or confusion. Some memory problems are serious, and others are not. If they are not, it is referred to as MCI (mild cognitive impairment). People who have serious changes in their memory, personality, and behavior may suffer from a form of brain disease called dementia. Dementia seriously affects a person's ability to carry out daily activities. Alzheimer's disease is one of many types of dementia.

My Symptoms	When they started	Frequency (circle)	Changes in frequency
I can't remember things		1 2 3 4	
I easily get confused		1 2 3 4	
I have trouble concentrating		1 2 3 4	
I have trouble learning things		1 2 3 4	
My brain does not work right		1 2 3 4	
I have a hard time understanding what people say to me		1 2 3 4	
(Other Symptoms)		1 2 3 4	
		1 2 3 4	
		1 2 3 4	
		1 2 3 4	

Frequency Scale: 1: never   2: occasionally   3: frequently   4: constantly

Problems with Thinking (Thought Disorders, Psychotic Disorders, Schizophrenia)

Thinking disorders, referred to as psychotic disorders are serious medical conditions resulting in problems with your ability to experience accurate thoughts, feelings, and sensations. You may hear sounds or voices or see images that others do not experience. You could also have beliefs and perceptions that are not accurate. Your thinking processes can be disorganized, racing, or blocked.

This condition can also lead to the following problems:

- Problems with thoughts about yourself and the environment.
- Difficulty talking to others.
- Suspicious of others or think someone is controlling your thoughts.
- Difficulty with lack of energy and interest in how you look.
- Learning concentration and problem-solving.

My Symptoms	When they started	Frequency (circle)	Changes in frequency
I hear or see things that are not real, or that others can't see or hear		1 2 3 4	
My thoughts are disorganized or confusing		1 2 3 4	
I hear voices telling me to do certain things		1 2 3 4	
I fear that others will harm me		1 2 3 4	
I think people are against me		1 2 3 4	
I find it hard to pay attention		1 2 3 4	
I have a hard time talking to others		1 2 3 4	
I don't like to be around others		1 2 3 4	
I don't like to do anything		1 2 3 4	
I don't care about my appearance		1 2 3 4	
(Other Symptoms)		1 2 3 4	
		1 2 3 4	
		1 2 3 4	

Frequency Scale: 1: never   2: occasionally   3: frequently   4: constantly

Problems with Sleep (Primary Sleep Disorder)

Primary sleep problems that result from:

- Difficulty getting to sleep or staying asleep.

- Difficulty having a restful sleep.

- The primary sleep problem causes significant distress in social, work, or other important areas of functioning.

- The sleep problem is not due to a medical condition.

My Symptoms	When they started	Frequency (circle)	Changes in frequency
I have difficulty getting to sleep		1 2 3 4	
I have difficulty staying asleep		1 2 3 4	
I do not have a restful sleep		1 2 3 4	
(Other Symptoms)		1 2 3 4	
		1 2 3 4	
		1 2 3 4	
		1 2 3 4	

Frequency Scale: 1: never   2: occasionally   3: frequently   4: constantly

Using Medication to Treat My Illness

Mental health medications are selected to treat your specific symptoms. Their purpose is to relieve your symptoms and provide better brain health. This process usually takes as least 4–6 weeks of regular dosage administration before they are able to improve the "communication system" in your brain. You will begin to see symptom relief when this happens. In order to obtain maximum relief for your symptoms, your must take your medication as prescribed by your doctor/nurse practitioner.

Possible side effects

There are side effects to all medications. Generally, mental health medication is safe and well-tolerated by most people. There are always risks and benefits to all medical treatment. Have your doctor and/or pharmacist explain the possible side effects for your medication. If you do experience side effects sometimes they are minor and will go away in a few days. Some are more difficult to tolerate and require a change of your medication and/or dosage.

If you experience any side effects report them to your doctor. If you decide to discontinue the medication, *please* discuss this decision with your doctor. Stopping some medications suddenly can cause serious side effects.

How to find the right medication

Sometimes it will take several trials of medication to find one that will work. You may need to take several medications to obtain maximum symptom relief. For example, you may have depression with anxiety, problems concentrating, and also have problems with energy and sleep. Your doctor may prescribe two different types of antidepressants or an antidepressant with another type of medication to get maximum relief of all your symptoms.

What are drug interactions?

It is *very* important that you are honest with your doctor and provide any information about all the medication you are taking or using as needed. Drug interactions can be very serious as well as interfere in the planned effects of your mental health medications or other prescribed medications.

Substances like nicotine, alcohol, caffeine, herbal medicine, and illicit drugs can also interfere in the metabolism or planned effects of your mental health medication. They also may cause serious reactions.

Paying for My Medications

If I have prescription drug insurance

It is very important that you are familiar with your health insurance and what benefits you have. Medication can be very expensive including some of the newer mental health medications. Most prescription plans require co-pays, which is your required amount to pay for each prescription.

Medications that have been manufactured for approximately 10 years are available in a generic form as well as a brand form. Generic medications usually cost less and have lower co-pay. Some prescription plans have a limit to the selection of mental health medications.

Have your doctor help you select medications that you can better afford and still provide the same relief.

If I do not have prescription drug insurance

If you need medication and do not have prescription drug insurance, please inquire into other means for obtaining your prescription. All medical problems are a concern, including mental health problems.

Ask your doctor the following questions:

1. Are there samples of the medication available for a limited time until other alternative payments can be explored?

2. Are there generic forms of medicine that are less expensive that you can afford?

3. Are there Patient Assistance Programs available to help provide the medication?

There are websites that have a complete list of patient assistant programs. One example is www.needymeds.com.

My Medication Plan

Date	Name of Medication	Dose	Number of Pills	When Taken	Symptoms Treated
				○ 1 each day (AM) (PM) ○ 2 times/day ○ 3 times/day ○ 4 times/day ○ at bedtime	
				○ 1 each day (AM) (PM) ○ 2 times/day ○ 3 times/day ○ 4 times/day ○ at bedtime	
				○ 1 each day (AM) (PM) ○ 2 times/day ○ 3 times/day ○ 4 times/day ○ at bedtime	
				○ 1 each day (AM) (PM) ○ 2 times/day ○ 3 times/day ○ 4 times/day ○ at bedtime	
				○ 1 each day (AM) (PM) ○ 2 times/day ○ 3 times/day ○ 4 times/day ○ at bedtime	

What are Possible Stumbling Blocks that Might Interfere With Taking My Medications?

Taking your medication correctly, sometimes referred to as medication compliance, is a very important partnership between you, your doctor and other members of your treatment team.

When you do not take your medications correctly, you do not get better. You may get sicker, and it can even worsen your medical condition. Most likely, you will have a relapse of your symptoms.

Reasons for medication noncompliance, according to research studies, are the following:

1. Patients do not understand their medical illness.

2. Patients want to use alcohol and street drugs.

3. Patients do not have a open therapeutic relationship with their doctor.

4. Patients are having side effects from the medication.

5. Patients are not seeing improvement in their symptoms.

6. Patients cannot afford the medication.

It is very important you are able to resolve any issues with your doctor that would prevent you from being compliant with your medications.

Ask yourself the following questions:

1. Do I tend to forget to take my medications?

2. When I feel good, do I sometimes not take my medications?

3. When the medication makes me feel worse or causes side effects, do I stop the medication without telling my doctor?

4. Do I tend to be disorganized and forgetful with my activities of daily living?

If you answer any of the above questions with "yes," you may be putting yourself at risk.

Other Possible Stumbling Blocks

Unhealthy Attitudes

Your friends or family may not understand the value of taking medications for your symptoms or they do not understand that mental illness is a medical problem like having heart problems. Sometimes you or your family may think that taking medication is a sign of weakness or feel embarrassed. You may want to talk to your doctor or your counselor about having them involved in your own education and understanding of your mental illness.

Other People's Opinions

Sometimes your friends and family want to give you "medical advice" that is not helpful or appropriate for you treatment. Your doctor or counselor is the best source of accurate information to understanding your illness and the treatment options available. Also check out information you may read or hear in the news media. The information may not be adequate for you to make informed decisions regarding your medications and treatment.

Taking Your Medication as Prescribed

It is important to understand how to take your medication and the times and dose to take. Work out the best times and methods with your doctor that suit your lifestyle. Use pillboxes or other routine reminders as a way to help. Request the best dosing method and time for you to remember. This is very important to get the maximum benefit of your medications.

Waiting For Your Medication to Work

Finding the right medication may take some time. The right medicine will also take time to work and make improvements in the chemical transmitters of your brain. This could take at least 4–6 weeks. You will see your symptoms gradually improve.

Safety

Keep you medicines in a safe and secure place. Do not share your medications with others or take medications not approved by your doctor. Take only the dose that is prescribed to you.

Annoying Side Effects

32

Discuss all side effects with your doctor. If the medication is working, there are ways to minimize or alleviate these side effects. Do not stop your medication on your own because of these side effects. Notify your doctor and discuss a plan to change or taper off the medication if the side effects are too uncomfortable.

Common Side Effects to My Mental Health Medications

1. Stomach or intestinal disturbances like nausea, constipation or diarrhea.

   Change what you eat or drink, have doctor lower the dose, change the time you take the medication, or change the medication.

2. Dizziness or drowsiness

   Your doctor may lower the dose if possible, change the time you take the medication, change the medication.

3. Dry mouth

   Use sugar-free gum or hard candy, or sipping water.

4. Sexual difficulties

   Your doctor may add an antidote medication or change the medication.

5. Weight gain

   Practice good nutritional habits with a low-fat, low-sugar diet, or switch to another medication. Always monitor your weight.

6. Skin rash, stiff joints, restlessness, feeling like a "zombie," or other serious side effects.

   Call your doctor immediately.

List the side effects you are having. Discuss them with your doctor.

MEDICATION	SIDE EFFECTS	SOLUTION

Helping to Prevent the Return of My Symptoms

What if my symptoms return?

Your medication is designed to help your symptoms gradually improve and to offer protection against the return of the symptoms. When you begin to feel better, keep taking your medications.

As long as you are taking your medications, your brain chemical transmitters will work more effectively. If you start to have symptoms again, your medication dosage may need to be increased. You are usually started on the lowest effective dose. You may require a higher dose for treating your symptoms. Everyone has differences on how the medication is metabolized in your body. Please call your doctor as soon as possible if your symptoms start to return.

If you stop taking your medication, your symptoms will most likely return. Relapse, or the return of your symptoms, would be painful and demoralizing. You also will likely have problems with work, relationship, or coping with problems in daily living.

Relapse, as you have learned, can cause additional problems for your brain health. The next time your brain may not respond as well the medications, your recovery will be longer, and you run the risk of not returning to normal functioning. It is similar to stopping your heart medication without discussing it with your doctor. You could cause your heart further damage.

Steps to prevent the return of my symptoms

To help prevent the return of your symptoms, follow these suggestions:

1. Develop an accurate understanding of you mental illness and how to best manage it.

2. Participate in your treatment plans, including attending your routine medication checks with your doctor and all your counseling/education sessions.

3. Take your medication as prescribed, appropriately manage side effects, and do not allow yourself to run out without have them refilled at the pharmacy.

4. Develop and practice healthier, more effective coping skills.

5. Keep track of your symptoms; if they worsen, report them immediately to your doctor.

On the following chart, make your own plan for preventing the return of your symptoms. You may want to include the suggestions already listed.

My Plan to Prevent the Return of My Symptoms

✔	MY PLAN
	1) Keep track of my symptoms
	2) Take my medication as prescribed
	3) Attend my appointments
	4) Complete homework assignments
	5) Eat at least 3 meals per day
	6) Sleep at least 6–8 hours at night
	7) Exercise 20–30 minutes a minimum of 3 times per week
	8) Reduce caffeine/nicotine intake and avoid alcohol or illicit drugs
	9) Structure my time to increase satisfaction and decrease stress
	10) Spend time with people that are supportive to my recovery and avoid people that might interfere with my recovery
	11)
	12)
	13)
	14)

Appendix

List of Mental Health Medications

Antidepressants

Medication	Brand Name	Condition(s) treated
amitriptyline	Elavil	Depression, pain, sleep
trazadone	Desyrel	Depression, sleep problems
fluoxetine	Prozac	Depression, premenstrual mood disorders, OCD
buproprian (SR/XL)	Wellbutrin (SR/XL)	Depression, smoking cessation, adjunct to Bipolar Rx, side effects for sexual dysfunction with SSRI's, sometimes ADHD
sertraline	Zoloft	Depression, panic disorder, premenstrual mood disorders, OCD
paroxetine	Paxil	Depression, panic disorder, premenstrual mood disorders, OCD
venlafaxine (XR)	Effexor XR	Depression, panic disorder
nefazadone	Serzone	Depression, panic disorder, premenstrual mood disorders
fluvoxamine	Luvox	Depression, panic disorder, OCD
mirtazapine	Remeron ST	Depression, panic disorder
citalopram/ escitalopram	Celexa/Lexapro	Depression, anxiety disorder
doloxetine	Cymbalta	Depression, chronic nerve pain

Medications for Thinking and Mood Disorders

Medication	Brand Name	Condition(s) treated
quetiapine	Seroquel	Thought disorder, symptoms of schizophrenia
halperidol	Haldol	Thought disorder, symptoms of schizophrenia
olanzapine	Zyprexa	Thought disorder, symptoms of schizophrenia, bipolar disorder
risperidone	Risperdal	Thought disorder, symptoms of schizophrenia, bipolar disorder
ziprasidone	Geodon	Thought disorder, symptoms of schizophrenia, bipolar disorder
lozapine	Loxitane	Thought disorder, symptoms of schizophrenia
aripiprazole	Abilify	Thought disorder, symptoms of schizophrenia

Medications for Mood Disorders

Medication	Brand Name	Condition(s) treated
lithium	Lithobid, Eskalith	Bipolar disorder, migraines, adjunct to thought an depressive disorders
carbamazapine	Tegretol	Bipolar, seizures, neuralgia pain
valproic acid	Depakote (ER)	Bipolar, seizures, adjunct to thought and depressive disorders
fluoxitane/ olanzapine	Symbyax	Bipolar, schizophrenia, and other thought disorders
oxcarbazepine	Trileptal	Bipolar disorders, seizures
lamotrigine	Lamictal	Bipolar disorders, seizures

Medications for Attention Problems

Medication	Brand Name	Condition(s) treated
amphetamine	Adderall, Adderall XL	ADD/ADHD, narcolepsy, depression that is not responding to antidepressants
methylphenidate	Ritalin, Concerta, Ritalin LA, Focalin CR	ADD/ADHD, narcolepsy, depression that is not responding to antidepressants
dextroamphetamine	Dexedrine	ADD/ADHD, narcolepsy, depression that is not responding to antidepressants
atomoxetine	Strattera	ADD/ADHD
modafinil	Provigal	Narcolepsy, fatigue in depression & MS, ADD/ADHD

Medications for Memory Problems

Medication	Brand Name	Condition(s) treated
donepezil	Aricept	Mild-moderate dementia, mild cognitive impairments
rivastigmine	Exelon	Mild-moderate dementia, mild cognitive impairments
memartine	Namanda	Moderate dementia
galantamine HBr	Reminyl	Mild-moderate dementia, mild cognitive impairments

Medications for Anxiety

Medication	Brand Name	Condition(s) treated
buspirone	Buspar	Anxiety
diazepam	Valium	Anxiety, relief of anxiety in depression
chlordiazepoxide	Librium	Anxiety, muscle relaxant, seizure disorder
oxazepam	Serax	Anxiety, ETOH W/D
clorazepate	Tranzene	Anxiety, ETOH W/D
lorazepam	Ativan	Anxiety, ETOH W/D
clonazepam	Klonopin	Anxiety, alcohol withdrawal acute mania, muscle spasms
alprazolam	Xanax (XR)	Anxiety, panic attacks

Medications for Sleep Problems

Medication	Brand Name	Condition(s) treated
flurazepam	Dalmane	Short term management of sleep problems
temazepam	Restoril	Short term management of sleep problems
triazolam	Halcion	Short term management of sleep problems
zolpidem	Ambien	Short term management of sleep problems
zalepon	Sonata	Short term management of sleep problems
espiclone	Lunesta	Long term management of sleep problems